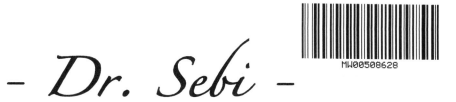
- Dr. Sebi -

Smoothie Detox Guide

7-Natural Ingredients to Rapid Body Detox.

31-Day Smoothies Plan with Affordable & Delicious Recipes

By **A. J. Bridgeford**

Book 5 of 7: of the series "Dr. Sebi's Natural Remedies"

About A. J. Bridgeford

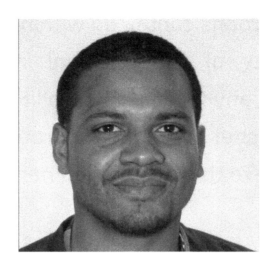

A.J. Bridgeford was born in South Africa and is an incredible traveler who has traveled the globe at least 10 times to discover the wonderful cultures belonging to various countries. His journey was interrupted when he lost his mother due to an unexpected and terrible illness. After this happened, he suffered a lot from depression until he realized that his mission was to find a solution to the most well-known diseases and help people in need. This research led him to Honduras, where he learned and practiced the revolutionary methodologies of the great Dr. Sebi. Since then, his mission has become to disseminate these incredible treatments and work in the field to improve people's lives. He is still fighting disease thanks to his private clinics with exceptional results. He wanted to bring back some of his most critical knowledge in the field of "alkaline-based medicine" with this book. With the wish for a healthier life, he reported a quote:

"Life is around us, and we are the fruit of life. Like any fruit, we need the natural elements that the earth makes available to us to become ripe and begin to new life".

Table of contents

Introduction

While our bodies occasionally have self-detox capability, they still send us clues that we should act from the outside. As the toxins arrive, our immune system, kidney, liver, and function get rid of it from the body. But as these contaminants surpass the body's ability to get rid of them, they are retained inside us for a lengthy period of time before appropriate action is taken out to fully get rid of them. You would never have to think about gaining weight if you simply adjust your dietary habits and fit with your body's normal capacity to heal, remain slim, and have energy. Several factors lead to weight gain, and toxic overload is one cause that is often underestimated by conventional diets.

Simply put, as bodies are loaded with contaminants, individuals also have trouble reducing weight. The further toxins you consume are subjected to each day, the more toxins you store in the body as fat cells. By dieting alone, toxins contained in fat cells are impossible to get rid of. You should detoxify your body first. The body shifts its energies away from eating calories when the body is overwhelmed with toxins and utilizes the energy to work faster to detoxify the body. Simply, the body can't consume calories, so as the body detoxifies and gets rid of toxins quickly, the energy will be used to lose fat. This is an incredible way in a really limited amount of time to change your wellbeing.

Dr. Sebi's diet has already shown that it has successfully improved the immune system, wellbeing, and raising energy. For a good and satisfying life, the liver is a really necessary organ as we should already realize, the way our liver works may be profoundly influenced by the type of food we consume. The secret to a safe, well-functioning liver is an easy and safe diet abundant in nutritious vegetables and fruits. So get prepared to take the initiative: Dr. Sebi 4 weeks Detox Smoothie plan.

Chapter 1 Introduction to dr. Sebi smoothies

The way to reduce weight, stay fit, look good, and enhance the quality of life is the smoothie diet, and it is a habit of drinking healthy smoothies every day.

It is something like a shift in your lifestyle that you never want to leave.

When you hear the term smoothie, the first thought that enters the mind is mason jars filled with mixed fruit and vegetables. And the vibrant mason jar content may taste great or may not, which is partially true.

Yeah, the so-called offers you the chance to drink kale, ginger, tomatoes, spinach, celery, carrots, some seasonal fruit. However, there's more, hence the belief that a lifestyle is smoothies drinking.

After the 1st and the 2nd day, mixing fruits with veggies and having smoothies daily become addictive.

Often, because you seasonally use fruits and vegetables, which relates to affordability, it is something that you can comfortably do on a regular basis, it becomes a routine.

Much of the time, you require a healthier and better formation than the previous one.

Even-time, the body calls for more, and you can't resist in addition to making the kitchen counter into a workspace for blending.

And compel your guests to test out whatever new smoothies' recipe you've come up with.

You soon learn that it is a routine to drink smoothies that keep offering.

Smoothies make you energetic; you can't stop wanting healthy food. The best thing is that when you're having fun, you reduce weight without trying.

A smoothie diet may not cause you to crave entire pizzas or burgers, unlike Keto, military, or Paleo diets (and any diet you may hear of), you only crave healthier foods.

Therefore, it is a safe lifestyle to drink smoothies every day.

It's not limiting, such as the lifestyle you desire, and unlike the diets you've pursued for decades, you can add in any vegetable and fruit in the blender. You can even throw nuts, powder, seeds, or spices.

We name it a smoothie diet and following a diet and sticking to it is the best way everyone stays healthy.

Instead of making you feel hungry, tired, and sick, you need a balanced lifestyle that helps you.

1.1 How long are you supposed to remain on a smoothie diet?

Do not think about this as a magical pill that would leave you looking healthier and slim in a week or days.

As long as you're around, you have to remain in the routine of having smoothies until you enjoy good health and want to keep a healthier weight.

In other terms, until the day when it begins sounding like a task, you have to cultivate this habit, and this becomes a routine.

Diets are scheduled to operate for a defined period of time, but it's timeless, much like having water, once you encounter a smoothie lifestyle.

Move your mind from why you are not losing weight quickly enough for the diet (smoothie lifestyle) to function, or is this getting me healthier?

Cleanses Smoothie

Although some weight is reduced by a 5 to 7-day smoothie cleanse, you will step out of it exhausted, and you would just cheat on unhealthier items.

1.2 The Diet Smoothie is Not really a Crash Diet

These crash diets contribute to extreme limits and starvation in calories.

Diets like smoothies don't.

While successful in the short period, crash diets have far more detrimental consequences, like metabolism that has been adversely affected.

The drastic steps slow down the metabolism and revving up is hard once the body adjusts to it, and you add weight quicker.

Lay down your long-term target before beginning a smoothie diet (it begins as a diet at least).

You will need a great connection with nutritious food.

A lifestyle smoothie improves metabolic activity to make it easier to lose weight.

one can still hold the weight off as long as one stick in the lifestyle of balanced eating

1.3 Smoothie Diet and Weight Loss All regarding eating healthy

A smoothie lifestyle emphasizes healthier food, as discussed above, and results in weight loss, improved health, and huge bursts of energy.

All on the plate should be nutritious and healthy for this diet to succeed.

And what's eating healthy?

Having a balanced diet is about healthy eating.

A balanced eating plan, according to the CDC, includes the below basics:

- Vegetables and fruits, milk goods that are low-fat/fat-free, and whole grain.

- Livestock, lean beef, beans, eggs, fish, plus nuts.

- And diets that are poor in saturated fats, trans fats, cholesterol, salt, and sugar supplements.

When they are not in season, you can still have canned or frozen vegetables and fruits.

Don't forget regarding foods high in calcium and keep under the regular calorie requirements.

You receive extra vitamins, but you get healthier by adding a smoothie in your regular meal plans.

1.4 How do smoothies help you really lose weight?

How are smoothies helping in the journey of weight loss?

Smoothies for weight reduction are lower in calories but higher in fiber and nutrients, curbing cravings for fatty foods, making you fuller for longer, & boosting digestive health.

Here are a few explanations for why smoothies are a very useful tool for weight loss:

Nutrient-dense are smoothies

Only think about all the natural vegetable and fruit vitamins and micronutrients in your cup now.

For various roles, all the smoothie's nutrients are absorbed by cells, and the outcome is well-developed cells, organs & body systems.

The smoothie's nutrients often mean that certain nutrients are not craved by the cells, and you are not going to turn to unhealthy foods to curb your cravings.

Do you realize that the shortage of nutrients is the product of a lot of the cravings?

And the cravings and crazy appetite can decrease by indulging in the nutrient-dense foods.

High micro-nutrient diets reduce the unpleasant consequences correlated with hunger, according to scientific research.

With an appetite as the greatest weight reduction impediment, it is of more value to rely on the number of nutrients you receive from food or drink compared to relying on the calorie intake.

A diet having high micronutrient helps in weight reduction and improved wellbeing in the long term.

Often, if you adhere to a diet of high micronutrients, the unpleasant mental and physical effects of hunger decrease.

So, you would have decreased headaches, stomach cramps, tremors, and attitude swings by having smoothies.

Further study suggests that body function and overall health are impaired by the consumption of harmful foods or foods deficient in dietary antioxidants, phytochemicals, and other important micronutrients.

This is because the aggregation of advanced glycation end products, lipid A2E, free radicals, lipofuscin that accumulate and raise inflammation, is induced by low micronutrient diets.

These goods render you more prone to obesity, as well.

Bottom line

For improved health and for weight control, you need nutrient-dense food such as smoothies.

You control your weight by managing your appetite.

Smoothies provide an easy way to make a healthier food regimen simpler.

A path of a million steps begins with one step, as the adage goes.

You will only meet your weight reduction objectives with the same thought by taking the first minor move, then several minor moves after the first one.

Instead of introducing hundreds of adjustments at once, implement minor dietary improvements In order to ease in a healthier lifestyle that contributes to weight reduction,

Make a health adjustment then warm it up to it before the next change is dropped.

Then you'll be far more inclined to adhere to the idea that the smoothie diet is easy and quick to implement into your everyday routine.

And, thus, can more efficiently lose and maintain the weight.

Weight reduction smoothies are enjoyable.

There is no other balanced food strategy that is as fun as a smoothie diet, contributing to weight loss.

You are free to put your favorite vegetables and fruit into your blender, as well as seeds, nuts, and herbs such as mint, and then drink all those rich flavors.

The result, all the time, surprises the taste buds of yours.

In the smoothies, there are also endless forms of masking the flavor of spinach or kale.

Your smoothie will help you experience good eating as long as you don't go crazy on the fruit.

Smoothies save your time because they are really easy to prepare.

If the limited time is the biggest explanation of why you can't lose weight, more smoothies need to be made.

Blending vegetables and fruit is a perfect and tasty alternative for the meals.

You don't have to excuse the shortage of preparation time and no preparation involved as the explanation behind the unhealthy cooking habits of yours.

Smoothies facilitate the control of calories.

You get better power over the calories when doing smoothies at home.

You can lose weight only because you eat more calories than you consume.

You will adjust the calorie count correctly as you find what fits better on your body.

You can use almond milk, coconut milk, or good old water instead of adding milk to your morning smoothie.

Bottom line

Since smoothies are delicious, nutrient-dense, save time, and are quickly blended into the diet, they are great for your path to weight loss or weight control.

By following the Smoothie Diet, how much weight will you lose?

They're healthy smoothies. But not all, smoothies. If you use the wrong ingredients, you can quickly transform the nutritious drink into a really unhealthy one. You get the impression of ice cream, chemical sweeteners (agave, honey, etc.), store-bought juice, yogurt, chocolate powder, chocolate syrup, pudding mix, whip, cold whip, soda cream. They are just going to undermine your attempts at weight reduction, so keep away from them. Often, you have to watch what you consume, with certain smoothies containing a number of calories, most getting more calories than the daily meal.

It depends on the kind of body you have

This suggests that on genetics, it may rely that the number of pounds you lose.

Some individuals lose weight quicker, naturally than others.

It relies on what (besides the smoothies) you consume.

You will lose extra weight if you consume nutritious meals and drink lots of water throughout the day than if you consume unhealthy, heavily unprocessed foods.

It depends on the activity level.

You can lose further weight if you exercise, go on walks, and visit the gym many days a week.

Yet the weight reduction path would be lengthy with plodding success if you're sedentary (unless extreme dietary changes made by you.)

Answer

Individuals normally lose 2-5lbs each week.

But even though that's the standard range We've seen, we know people who, during their 1st week, dropped 20 pounds.

What we can guarantee you, though, is this:

You Can see results if you proceed with the smoothie diet.

Chapter 2 The natural ingredients to rapid body detox

There are different meanings of phrases and words, such as detox. It may imply anything not made by humans (an animal, a plant) or a substance with no added additives (herbal medicine, organic food), among its multiple meanings. For you, detox does not necessarily mean healthy.

There's detox too, To eliminate toxins and encourage overall health, it has a purpose in respect to eating natural food. It even has another category to initial treatment use disorders like drug abuse and alcoholism.

Important it knows that what you'll need.

2.1 Detoxification, what is it?

Detoxification is the cleaning of unidentified body contaminants (toxins) and also the exclusion of body intoxicants (opioids, drugs, alcohol) until participation in something like a SUD (substance use disorders) or recovery program from addiction. They aren't the exact thing.

Uniform Alcoholism & intoxication Care Act (1971) suggested that better it was for those with an AUD (alcohol use disorders) to undergo medication instead of prosecution, detoxification became standard procedure for people with AUD (alcohol use disorder). They might "lead regular lives as citizens of the community" in that manner.

2.2 What Detox Do?

For detox working, you should avoid utilizing or having a harmful substance that triggers your health issues, including lead-containing materials, fatty foods, or addictive things like alcohol or narcotics. Then the liver, digestive system, kidneys, lungs, and skin of your body remove the residual contaminants, taking the body back to its pre-toxin condition. The body normally needs time if it's healthy.

Some individuals claim that with an intense diet, you will speed up the Process, vigorously eliminating the toxins: supplements (natural), juicing foods, or proprietary tonics for best digestion.

2.3 Detox Full Body

In the common context, a cleanse or complete body detox is a way to purge the body "toxins" (chemicals and impurities and pollutants) to stay healthy to live happy and longer.

As long as you're healthy, drinking healthy fluids, and sufficient water and eating good food, then this detox type is what our body is actually prepared to do it without any support. It's a diet, in fact. Involving vegetables and Juicing fruits, taking away toxic things (coffee, sugar, tobacco, alcohol), and exercise.

If you eat vegetables and fruits instead of refined grains, beef, sugar, and wheat, you'll lose weight, get more stamina, and feel better, so you don't have to drink those juices. You should enjoy vegetables and fruit. Good for you is the food fiber. It is needless to juice food or purchases pricey juices containing dietary supplements.

2.4 Detoxing Misconceptions

Detox is a normal step in a balanced body and does not need attention. You will get fewer chemicals in your system once you avoid eating them, although there is no proof that diet programs quick up the method. If you have lesser toxins in the body, you are going to accumulate lesser toxins. Few popular misconceptions regarding detoxifying involve:

- Using detox techniques would not accelerate the removal of contaminants from the system. All the so-called contaminants are not named, and there is no proof of any contaminants exiting the body sooner due to detox.

- Detox regimes do not help you shed weight. Yeah, once you avoid consuming sugars, fried products, and carbs, you are likely to lose fat; however, you are losing food, not pollutants. When you take diuretics and laxatives, you can lose weight throughout the near term, but it is because you are running to the toilet many times. You may end up becoming dehydrated dangerously.

- Activated charcoal would not flush out liquor. It is utilized for purifying or aeration in manufacturing operations. Some also reported this to purify and avoid or ease cramps or even excessive drinking.

Worse still, one contaminant that charcoal cannot flush off is liquor. It may inhibit the ingestion of many other compounds, but it may be the nutrients that you require.

2.5 Colonic Irrigation and Colon Cleansing

Another component of full-body detoxification includes emptying the colon of stools built up and bacteria, either by colon cleansing (laxative-rich elixir) or by flushing water in gallons (colonic irrigation).

These techniques have their own assumptions like

- You do not have 40 lbs of intestine fecal matter. It is more of an lb, and there is no indication that it must be extracted any quicker than the body's normal processes let.

- Colonics do not make you drop weight. Although you may drop 1-2 pounds in the short run, methods may create side effects (undesirable and harmful).

- Colon-cleaning treatments do not extract colon lining bacteria. It is not essential; the colon line cells are shed and then replaced every 3 days. And if it's appropriate, not all body bacteria can be dangerous. We require some of them for better health.

That does not mean that there is no advantage of a full detox; it is just that they're not physical. They may be physiological or spiritual. It could be related to the observer's effect: when you are striving to do best, you are feeling better. It is not bad once in a year what research on detox diets is focused almost entirely on animals. Good liver and kidneys are far more essential than overpriced supplements and juices.

2.6 Detox Drug / Alcohol

Alcohol and drug detoxification is a severe medicinal procedure. It includes turning away from narcotics or alcohol and eventually learning to avoid. It is a lot riskier and more complicated since these drugs rewire the brain of yours, so without them, you cannot work. You may naturally detoxify the alcohol or narcotics amount you consume, or even avoid eating cold turkeys, although it could be dangerous. Alcohol and medications may be physically and psychologically harmful. When you avoid using these, you can suffer signs of withdrawal: cold sweating, trembling of your hands, vomiting and nausea, and problems of the heart. You might think you are going to fail and begin using it again. Symptoms like these may last for a few months. In serious addiction, especially alcohol & benzodiazepines (Valium, Xanax), quitting cold turkey may be catastrophic. Nelsan Ellis, the actor of True Blood, died when he struggled to escape drinking independently, culminating in infection of the blood, lower blood pressure, swelling liver, and heart and kidney failure. It is important crucially that before you begin to detoxify yourself and at home, you get medical advice.

Drug or liquor detoxifying approaches

At least there are three forms of withdrawal for SUD (substance use disorders)

• Natural. Non-medical detox is also referred to as the social paradigm, through which you eventually avoid consuming the product or completely quit utilizing that without medicinal help. Fasting, hydration, and fitness (herbal remedies, water, teas, & juices) could be used.

• Medicinal detoxification of a human. Often referred to as the treatment paradigm, which is also close to naturally detox, only that qualified health care practitioners can efficiently handle the life-threatening side effects. Pulse rhythm, heart rate, & the breath shall be controlled. This detox can also require the usage of pain meds & medication-assisted care or substitutes (buprenorphine, methadone) at least before complete is the withdrawal, and you are eligible for rehabilitative care. Doctors also prescribe Vivitrol (opioid antagonists naltrexone) to keep people from being addicted if they relapse aftercare.

• Fast detoxification. Often known as AAROD (anesthesia-assisted rapid/fast opiate detoxification) or UROD (ultra-fast opioid detoxification), rapid detoxification accelerates the withdrawal process and restricting it to 3 days or less. The procedure requires an opioid blocker (naloxone naltrexone) to reverse the impact of any narcotics present inside and to put the person under medication for around 6 hours while the worst withdrawal effects. Regrettably, the procedure is risky than utilizing buprenorphine, which is also unpleasant and no longer effective. The united states Alcohol Community maintains that the method also isn't suggested.

2.7 Process of detoxing

When the person chooses or chooses to go through rehab for opioid use dependency, the phase of detoxification starts. Detox, therefore, is not the first stage. There are 3 main stages: assessment, stabilization, then fostering. They demonstrate the person, among other aspects, that everyone cares for them, their healing, recovery, and wellness.

- **Assessment.** No two addictions are precisely similar, and no human also. The formulation of a successful opioid addiction recovery strategy includes a thorough evaluation of the client's medication usage to ascertain whether there're any co-occurrence conditions (bipolar disorder, trauma, tension, depression, anxiety) that may have contributed to or worsened SUD. The assessment helps the customer and the workers to leave the field after the detox has been accomplished.

- **Stabilization**. This involves actual recovery while also training the client — including others near to them, friends, and families— for what occurs in recovery after detoxification is full. A stable support structure is an integral aspect of the long-term healing phase.

- **Fostering**. It is not sufficient for the individual to choose to undergo care or also to initiate care. They have needed to complete treatment. Alone detox is a temporary cure. If individuals may not learn to manage without drugs or liquor if they do not fix the problems that lead to substance addiction, & if they may not have ongoing support, addiction and another detox need are much possible.

A non-legally binding care arrangement is often enough to hold patients centered on true rehabilitation, not a brief respite.

2.8 Finest Instant Detox Foods

The positive news is that your kidneys and liver do a really good job of cleaning your body without consuming weird concoctions, juices, or fasts. And some tasty foods with excellent slimming and detoxification properties are there, which includes tea, which helps you lose 10 pounds. Hold the cayenne and vinegar, cleanse the pounds without any torture with the initial plan's help,—and the tasty foods below.

Grapefruit

Instead of revising the whole diet to tone down for the New Year, all you need to do is just consume some grapefruit before any meal. According to a study reported, this strategy will help you slash the middle by up to 1 inch. The researchers relate the heavy results to the fatting phytochemicals of the grapefruit. However, the fruit may interfere with some drugs adversely, so consult with the doctor before eating.

Bananas

No matter how much rounded your belly really is, your abs will be banished from view by bloat. Fortunately, one of the incredible stuff bananas bring to the body is to battle back against water loss and gas. According to studies published in the journal Anaerobe, consuming the fruit twice daily as a pre-meal snack will minimize tummy-bloat by fifty percent. Bananas have two magic powers to make the belly trim down: they improve the stomach to fight with bloat and have a good potassium dose that will help decrease water loss.

Spinach

To drive away hunger automatically, all you should do is to include some lettuce in your meal. The green fibers via an Appetite report include a potent hunger reducing compound named thylakoids. One of the best facts about spinach is that it has very minimum calories. Well, move forward and adds that in your morning smoothie, breakfast omelet, or sandwich for lunch to top up.

Mustard

One of the strongest ingredients to improve your Metabolism is probably lying inside everyone's refrigerator, and that's none other than mustard. According to researchers at Britain's Oxford Polytechnic University, consuming only one teaspoon of mustard for a mere 5 calories will improve the Metabolism with up to 25 percent for many hours. Smear some spread on a turkey sandwich. You can even consume it as a meat marinade. So consuming protein also burn your calories.

Sweet Potatoes

Suppose you feel a little pasty in winter, roast a few sweet potatoes. With carotenoids, you get such a sun-kissed skin tone, as it is a natural substance that gives the potato cubes that orange shade. Only twice the average of a normal potato with skin contains 200 percent of the permissible regular consumption of carcinoids, so eat up.

Beets

Although we wouldn't suggest a tough-core, nutrition-free detox for New Year's, we can provide a tactic just adding those ordinarily-detoxifying beets in your bowl. These gem-toned roots have a type of antioxidant that helps restore and rebuild liver cells, the main detox core of the body, and that is known as betalains. Your liver can feel overworked if you're already trying to keep warm. Beets are going to offer it a little boost, and then you're primed for the full party season coming spring.

Wild Salmon

Add a piece of salmon if you are going to quit smoking as a resolution for New Year. A balanced diet high in omega-3 fatty acids will help counteract arterial stiffness, a typical risk factor of smoking blocks blood cleaning flow via the vital organs and arteries, claim by Penn State scientists. A three-week analysis in Cardiology's article showed that those smokers having an intake of 2 grams of omega-3s a day saw a significant change in arteries' stiffness, facilitating balanced blood flow what you can see in a 4-ounce piece of salmon.

Lemon water

Begin creating a water-filled big pitcher with sliced lemons every day, and drinking at least up to eight glasses before going to bed. While no systematic research has correlated detoxification with lemon, it is important for a balanced working metabolism. You give the body the power needed to cleanse of contaminants while you intake water.

Collard Greens

A traditional crop of South cuisine, which is collard greens, particularly when boiled, has an amazing potential to purify your body with unnecessary cholesterol. The bile acid-binding ability of steamed collard greens was linked to Cholestyramine, a cholesterol-minimizing medication, in a new study reported in the journal Nutrition Science. Unbelievably, eating collards strengthened the body's cholesterol-obstruct mechanism to 13 %, far more than medication.

Asparagus

Ask the staff for a piece of steamed asparagus while you're having a tray of greasy dining fare, praying the Hangover Lord for mercy. As per a report published in Food Science, minerals and amino acids present in asparagus can relieve hangover indication and defend liver cells from toxins. The vegetable spears, too, are purely diuretic and can help rid the bloodstream with unnecessary toxins.

Turmeric

You may place an ice pack over your stabbing brain, but order the curry to have the exact anti-inflammatory benefit all over the rest of the body. Analysis suggests that curcumin, a chemical extracted mostly from the shiny-orange spice turmeric, acts in the liver as an effective anti-inflammatory. Research in the Gut journal showed that curcumin supplementation could substantially minimize the bile duct blockage and curved scarring if interacted with chemical processes associated with an inflammatory reaction.

White Tea

You can calm your nerves by drinking whatever tea you like, but white tea can easily help you in your weight loss with a little amount, and its even a part of The 7-Day Flat-Belly Tea Cleanser. The research reported in the journal Nutrition and Metabolism demonstrated that white tea increases lipolysis (fat breakdown) and obstruct adipogenesis (fat cell formation) at the same time. The caffeine and epigallocatechin-3-gallate (EGCG) mixture of tea appears to set fat cells up for the loss.

Guacamole

Think about guacamole as an appointed driver for the digestive system. The research included in The Journal of Agricultural Food Chemistry studied the results of feeding 22 separate fruits to rats with liver damage induced by galactosamine, a liver toxin. You assumed: avocado. Cilantro, the flavorful herb that offers guac its typical flavor, includes a special oil blend that sends the message of "simmer down" to the upset tummy. In fact, patients suffering from IBS (irritable bowel syndrome) relief with cilantro, as per a research published in the international Digestive Diseases and Sciences.

Hibiscus Tea

For sure, you must have put on so much weight if you have been drinking soup trying to keep yourself all warm, and as a result, your clothes may tighten up. Cheer up. Most probably, there's no weight gain if you just stick with a very healthy diet full of nutrients; you're just blown-up due to salty broths. There will be a paunchy tummy if there's sodium consumption very much as the body absorbs fluids. Fortunately, the remedy is simple: drink hibiscus tea. This will help in the shrinking of your tummy.

Tomatoes

Eating foods rich in antioxidants such as tomatoes will help avoid skin harm from inside out. In one British Journal of Dermatology research, research participants who consumed five tbsp of tomato sauce a day had 33% more defense from sunburn than the control group. There's nothing to worry about. You can just go down straight. For a boost of Mediterranean taste, searching for lower-sodium variations to hold bloating at bay & adding it to omelets, sauces, soups, or stews is the best thing one can do.

Detox Water

Can you guess a very quick way to shape your tummy, and for that, you don't even have to waste your time counting calories, spending your entire day at the gym, or just trying out the new trend to shape you up? Well, you got it: Detox water. When making efforts to have a healthy body, sweating the snacks and stress away seems great for sure.

But you know that annoying weight of the water can stick to your tummy through the cleanest day of eating and the most passionate workout session, and that's when you need nothing but fruit water. It's no surprise that gulping regular H2O may be less than relaxing, but there are enjoyable ways to render this good routine with less hassle. Some fruits have detoxifying characteristics inside them; cut them whole into your drink to enjoy the benefits and reach your water intake limit with an injection of taste.

Cocoa Powder

There's really great news for all those chocolate lovers out there. You don't have to worry about gaining weight or quieting chocolate as Cocoa powder, especially the unprocessed raw one, brings more fiber to your daily routine diet. All you have to do for a healthy diet is take two tablespoons of cocoa powder and mix it into hot water. This ensures that you are having the best diet as it contains 4 g of fiber.

Blackberries

A cup of blackberries(antioxidant-rich), which are packed in 7.6 g of fiber, is best. By mixing both of them, you trigger the gut to produce fatty acid butyrate, which lowers fat-causing inflammation in your body. The researchers found that all those having diets enriched with insoluble fiber contain higher amounts of ghrelin — which is an appetite-controlling hormone. Shed pounds quickly in mins and easily — by cooking these necessary, tasty, and tested recipes for oats that assist with weight loss.

Sunflower Seeds

Just a cup of one quarter sunflower seeds contains only over 200 Cals and contains 3g of fiber; also, sunflower seeds create a healthy and satisfying addition to every diet, offering magnesium a reasonable share, a mineral which holds regular the blood pressure, retains stable heart rhythm & helps improve lipolysis, a mechanism through which fat is released by the body from its reserves. Consider mixing them onto salads and oatmeal if you want extra crunch.

Oats

A rich type of gut-friendly fiber is called oats. One cup of oats contains 16 g of fiber, which includes insoluble fiber that feeds your intestine with harmful bacteria, and a soluble form named beta-glucan. Bonus: Oats also include avenanthramide, an anti-inflammatory agent that tests indicate may help to reduce health issues linked with obesity, including cardiac diseases such as diabetes. And a study in the American College of Nutrition Journal shows that oatmeal in the cereal aisle can be the most filling snack, resulting in stronger and long-lasting satiety emotions than ready-to-eat breakfast cereal.

Legumes

Although it may seem counterintuitive to consume anything that will help you to lose weight, it's really a good plan. Researchers observed in a four-week analysis reported in the European Journal of Nutrition that research participants who consumed a calorie-restricted diet with four weekly legume servings lost weight than those people who were on a calorie-equivalent diet which did not involve beans, possibly due to the high fiber content of the legume. Add chickpeas, lentils, tomatoes, and beans to enjoy the rewards at home in your weekly diet. Those were the same varieties of legumes in the sample that the researchers consumed.

Artichokes

For your buddy's spring wedding, you went out on a whim and purchased a snug little outfit, one size too short. Now for the fact you need to get slim in a month and a half, don't panic. Here's the strategy: rather than overhauling the whole meal, just include artichoke in your dinner salad. According to Wake Forest University researchers, in each 10 g of fiber you consume every day, your middle may bear 3.7 percent fewer flab. Only one artichoke will assist you in hitting the day's nutritious mark — and appear slim as ever on your buddy's special day.

Almonds

Drinking those winter drinks leaves you worse than overweight and hungover; you are at elevated risk of liver cancer because of the fatty compounds that build up in your liver subsequent days of overeating and drinking. However, according to a recent report by the British Journal of Nutrition, just a few tiny handfuls of vitamin-packed almonds a day could help clean the deposits and lower levels of "poor" LDL cholesterol.

Cold Potatoes

In case you ordinarily eat the potatoes warm, you are lost out on the spud's extra fat-fighting ability. When the potatoes are cooked & cooled within the fridge, its edible starches turn to safe starches through retrogradation. The body should work more to process safe starch, which advances fat oxidation & abdominal fat is reduced. If the thought of consuming cold spuds isn't inviting, consider utilizing them to create a potato serving of mixed greens. Enable them to cool after baking the red potatoes or Yukon

Gold and then break them into tiny pieces. Decorate them up fresh pepper, Dijon mustard, dill, sliced green onions, and simple Greek yogurt. And add it all together and place it to cool in the fridge before feeding.

Kiwi

In case you have got bowels or endure incessant obstruction. You must have heard that including fiber to the diet might be supportive, and you might not be aware that only some supplement sources are as viable as kiwi. IBS (Irritable Bowel Disorder) Patients with who ate 2 kiwis once a day for a whole month had constipation less and a common reduction of IBS side effects than the ones who didn't in a research conducted by Taiwanese analysts. Include the effective natural product to your oats, toss it into the smoothies or mix it with fruits in reviving salad.

Chapter 3 Advantages of smoothies, 4 weeks smoothies challenge and Recipes.

3.1 Advantages of smoothies

Other than weight reduction, there are Far more advantages involved with consuming vibrant smoothies.

Below are the advantages of the smoothie diet:

Losing weight and maintaining weight

You know that already, but, really, if you're searching for a quick way to reduce weight, then go no farther than the green smoothies.

Detox the body

Certain people think smoothies as detoxifying agents, and they're not mistaken. But again, to maximize detoxification, you need to guarantee that the smoothie contains all the necessary ingredients. As they are high in antioxidants, vegetables and fruits are detoxifying agents naturally.

In fruits and vegetables, antioxidants neutralize free radicals.

Free Radicals cause oxidative stress.

Inflammation of cells is caused by oxidative stress; inflammation induces disorders such as cancer and cardiac diseases.

How do you boost your smoothies' detoxification ability?

You should add ingredients such as Matcha tea in your smoothies, in addition to the vegetables and fruits in season.

As they are also high in antioxidants, you can also incorporate ingredients like fresh blueberries, kale, and grapes.

Garlic, papaya, and beets are other detoxifying ingredients of smoothie worth noting.

This increases cleaning and also boost the capacity of the liver to remove toxins efficiently.

But here's the best thing of smoothie detoxification-you get to speed up your body metabolism and drop weight even more easily.

You are kept hydrated by smoothies

The vegetables and fruit in the smoothies contain, primarily, water and fiber.

Therefore, you edge closer to the required regular water uptake through consuming smoothies.

The meal you take also offers water.

The other explanation of why smoothies overtook coffee as our preferred beverage is the hydration feature of smoothies.

You eat fewer, and for longer, you remain fuller.

You need energy from food, but this is an unlikely wish for humans; smoothies bring this likelihood similar to reality.

The making of smoothies, the mixing that takes place after the vegetables and fruits are washed and sliced, leaves you with such a nutrient-dense drink filled with nutrients.

For longer, the fibers hold you full.

Not every smoothie has the power to make you comfortable.

Avocados, for example.

Not only can avocados make devilishly dense and extremely delicious smoothies, but they also leave you happy for longer.

There are more protein and fiber in avocados than any other known fruits.

Two-in-one advantages: you no longer tend to eat unhealthy sweets through remaining satisfied for longer, and weight reduction occurs naturally.

Fight cravings for junk & genuinely want nutritious foods

Uncontrolled appetite is the cause of increasing cases of overweight and obesity.

We consume most of the time because hormones misinterpret the incorrect signs, not because we're starving.

You get to consume fewer if you can manage how hungry you are.

Smoothies hold you complete for a longer period, as described above.

As a consequence, when you are starving, you need less sugar and heavily processed food that your body demands.

You can't have any smoothie in order for this to function.

Fruits and vegetables, and even more proteins, are full of filling & fat-burning smoothies.

As described above, avocado is a protein-rich fruit that is incredibly filling.

But it's not the only source of proteins.

Try cottage cheese, almonds, Greek yogurt, and hemp protein for non-avocado fans for those in search of an alternative.

Apart from the protein filling, how about spinach?

Spinach also has thylakoids that decrease the appetite.

What are the functions of Ghrelin & leptin hormones in appetite and hunger control?

Leptin is a hormone that suppresses appetite, and ghrelin is the screamer of appetite.

There are elevated ghrelin levels and depressed leptin receptors in people suffering from and dealing with obesity.

The consumption of smoothie's protein-rich is essential in order to regulate cravings.

Protein-rich diets decrease postprandial ghrelin levels, contributing to a reduced appetite, according to research.

The high-protein diet impairs the insulinotropic polypeptides glucose-dependent that mediate ghrelin responses.

In comparison, a protein-rich smoothie delays gastric emptying by prolonging the sensation of fullness, which suppresses ghrelin release and raises the concentrations of leptin in fat cells.

Increase the intake of fruit & vegetables

You ought to consume 5 to 9 servings of vegetables & fruits every day for outstanding fitness and disease prevention.

The American Cancer Society states that it is important for treating several other disorders and cancer.

The notion of eating vegetables and fruits isn't appetizing, but smoothies are enticing.

Thus, green smoothies offer a fast and easy way to ensure that you consume your fruits and dark, leafy vegetables without needing to chew them.

You can consume more vegetables and fruit, as the fruits hide the flavor and the vegetables' scent.

Think of kale and spinach with strawberries, mangoes, pineapples, apples, and bananas

The best part of your regular smoothie is getting 3 - 5 (or sometimes more) fruit and vegetable servings.

Nutrition-boosting smoothies

The alternate title for smoothies should be a nutrient-bursting beverage.

In this book, most of the smoothies leave you with 100 % of the daily recommended intake of nutrients.

With the exception of vitamins B12, K, C, E, and folate, smoothies have more than adequate vitamin A (beta-carotene) and B vitamins.

Minerals such as calcium, magnesium, phosphorus, manganese, iron, copper, potassium, and trace elements are also obtained.

Since blending the vegetables and fruit breaks down plant cells, enhancing their digestibility, you get all these minerals and vitamins.

Blending also activates the complete capacity of vegetables and fruits, optimizing nutrient transfer to the body.

Enhanced digestion

Your overall wellbeing is decided by gut health, as Hippocrates stated: "all diseases originate in the gut."

You will regain your digestive health when a stressed lifestyle wreaks havoc on the digestive system of yours.

Your gut's health plays a vital role in the wellness of your immune system and digestive systems since the healthy bacteria in the gut control the body's ability to consume minerals and vitamins.

The bacteria also influence hormone control, vitamin output, digestion, immune responses, toxin removal, and mental health.

Your digestive tract also contains the enteric nervous system, the second brain.

Therefore, the wellbeing of the gut needs to be maintained in great condition.

The digestive tract's wellbeing is of fundamental significance, with medical disorders such as irritable bowel syndrome, intestinal hyperpermeability, and celiac disease correlated with general health concerns and psychiatric problems such as depression.

Green smoothies boost digestive wellbeing owing to the abundance of nutrients and fiber.

Fiber strengthens bowel motions. For bad bacteria, a clean bowel is an undesirable breeding site.

The clear bowel often increases the absorption of nutrients. Fiber, thus, is important for the health of the colon and gut.

In addition, the smoothie's nutrients feed the helpful gut microbes, helping in optimal digestion and a healthy immune system.

Great Immunity

When it doesn't have to be in a relentless battle with inflammation, the immune system functions well.

A healthy lifestyle leaves the body full of free radicals that cause cells to suffer from oxidative stress, inflammation, and damage.

Safe and antioxidant-enrich smoothies neutralize free radicals.

The consequence is the immune system doesn't get weak all the time to combat inflammation and infections.

Antioxidants improve immune function.

Apart from berries, sweet potatoes may be added to your smoothies.

Sweet potatoes, due to their abundance in beta-carotene, go beyond increasing flavor by strengthening the immunity.

For your bones and teeth, sweet potatoes are perfect.

Helps to reduce levels of blood cholesterol

Diets Plant-based are successful in reducing bad cholesterol and elevated cholesterol blood levels.

The smoothie diet embrace appears to have changed it around, aside from taking out harmful fats and heavily refined foods.

Sleep is easier

We hardly have time to relax owing to countless commitments, and then when we've time, insomnia is nearby.

It's time to find a permanent cure, and smoothies can help, as sleep is important for creativity, weight loss, health, healthy skin, and a positive mood.

Smoothies are high in ingredients (magnesium and calcium) that boost your sleep, in addition to cleansing your system, keeping the body in outstanding health.

Since they are high in calcium and magnesium, bananas, kiwis, and oats are excellent sleeping aids.

The tryptophan usage in the brain is facilitated by calcium.

To synthesize the melatonin, a sleep-inducing hormone, you need tryptophan.

For deep sleep, magnesium is vital as well.

Elevated amounts of energy

Smoothies offer you an extreme boost in vitamins.

Amongst other nutrients, you even get antioxidants and minerals that boost digestive function.

A digestive system bogged down dampens your morale, thus throwing your level of energy below zero.

However, when you consume nutritious smoothies, the immune system functions properly, your digestive tract's efficiency, and the absorption of nutrients increases.

These leave you with a burst of energy.

Smoothies are high in vitamins B and magnesium that promote energy metabolism.

Often, because you sleep well, you'll have more stamina all day long.

Bones Stronger

Bone-building necessities, smoothies ideally strengthen the resilience of your muscles and teeth as an ideal source of nutrients such as calcium, magnesium, and phosphorus.

Vitamin K in smoothies, in addition to calcium, is useful for avoiding brittle bones.

Broccoli, spinach, and many other green leafy vegetables contain vitamin K.

Clean, beautiful skin, healthier hair, and nails

'Though makeup helps you look beautiful and keeps blemishes from showing, the acne or other skin disorder, but they don't resolve the cause of it.

Smoothies leave skin with a flawless, young-looking, and radiant complexion by ridding the system of yours of chemicals, cleaning the digestive tract, and making you sleep easier.

For the production of collagen, vitamin C is important in smoothies.

For the elasticity of the skin and the firm look, collagen is the required protein.

The fine lines, the wrinkles are often faded away by smoothies.

And how about your hair?

Well, smoothies are high in vitamins and minerals that are important for hair strength and growth.

The introduction of proteins into your smoothies often provides you with adequate amino acids required for keratin production.

Yeah, smoothies even boost the protection of your nails.

Boosts the function of the brain

In smoothies, the nutrients have brainpower improving abilities.

The nutrients boost the brain's efficiency, providing you with a greater degree of mental awareness and attention.

Smoothies tend to be stronger than coffee-having no side effects, also no slump in the afternoon.

You may add certain elements rich in omega-3 fatty acids, such as coconut, for improved brain activity.

Lessens Depression Symptoms

There is a growing amount of people all over the world suffering from depression.

With all the current studies on how to ease the effects of depression, folate is one of the foods that tend to alleviate depression.

The addition of vegetable folate-rich into the smoothies would also help to improve your mood.

Folic acid Great sources include broccoli, peas, bananas, citrus fruits, and spinach.

Relieving seasonal allergies

While on a smoothie diet, the seasonal intensity of allergies decreases.

Those allergies that were at some point intolerable are now managed and less serious.

Smoothies aid In the treatment of pre & post-menopausal problems

Getting older makes you smarter, but it also allows you to be vulnerable to osteoporosis and heart disease.

Our smoothie diet, having done thorough studies, would allow our move to menopause even more tolerable.

Smoothies, especially flaxseed-rich ones, relieve menopausal symptoms.

Phytoestrogens (lignans) have an estrogenic influence on flax seeds.

When you reach menopause, estrogen levels fall, and the result, among other symptoms, is hot flashes.

While flaxseeds phytoestrogens do not meet the usual estrogen content, hot flashes are decreased by flaxseeds.

In reducing the effects of menopause, calcium is also important.

Smoothies improve the intake of calcium

For different body functions, including maintaining strong and healthy bones and teeth, you require calcium.

But this isn't it, calcium is important for blood clotting, control of the heart's rhythm, and nerve impulses transmission.

Although about 99 percent of calcium is contained in the teeth and bones, the body tissues and blood provide the remaining 1%, thus the need for supplementation.

Since they have strong calcium sources, you could add dark leafy vegetables and dried beans to your smoothies.

Ideal fiber source

The optimum fiber consumption suggested is between 25 – 30 gm.

When you have to push yourself to eat vegetables, consuming all this fiber is difficult.

You get further fiber, just like nutrients, by mixing vegetables and fruits and having smoothies.

From the blended vegetables and fruits, you get insoluble fiber.

Apples, avocados, pears, oranges, and berries are among the insoluble fiber best sources.

Enhances and protects vision

The four most common antioxidants present in smoothies are Beta-carotene, lutein, zeaxanthin, and resveratrol.

As smoothies are hydrating, they shield the eyes from dehydration also eyestrain.

For good eye protection, vitamin A and beta-carotene from the smoothies are essential.

Lutein and Zeaxanthin are commonly present in the retina and also in the lens.

It is known that these two carotenoid substances have defensive effects. They also will the chance that you may have cataracts.

Resveratrol, which is present in grapes, is an antioxidant that protects the body from skin conditions correlated with age, such as macular degeneration.

Smoothies inhibit the growth and persistence of chronic illnesses

How the body responds to diseases is determined by nutrition, diet, and lifestyle.

You reduce the chances of acquiring diseases like type II diabetes, obesity, cardiovascular disease, and cancer by adopting a healthier lifestyle.

Smoothies defend against arthritis, gout, and allergies, Alzheimer's disease, fibromyalgia, multiple sclerosis, lupus, stroke, and Parkinson's disease in conjunction with a healthy diet.

Since smoothies have antioxidants that battle free radicals, all these advantages come in.

The smoothies often improve digestive wellbeing, curbing medical problems arising from bad health of the gut.

More explanations of smoothies are important

- They are super simple to make & clean up.

- They taste deliciously heavenly.

- They are digestible easily.

- They are the ideal drink.

- An infinite range of recipes.

- They're pretty fun to make.

- And most of all: your mood is lifted.

We have found that you feel better immediately, and your mood improves just by adding more vegetables and fruit into the lifestyle.

Over the years, many celebrities have come up with ideas for smoothies. A large number of celebrities' drink smoothies for weight reduction and weight control at the same time.

There has been some influence in the smoothies the celebrities consume and the recipes they post or offer, though we don't know a lot about their lifestyles.

So, smoothies are transforming lives.

And now, when you have completely understood the reason behind it, let's dig into the way it's done.

3.2 Extra tips for the success of the weight loss and smoothie lifestyle

The smoothie diet will be difficult in the beginning, and we would not want you to quit halfway.

Before you whet the hunger for the smoothie diet, these extra tips will guarantee that you have what you need to know to maximize your attempts to lose weight.

Stick with this diet for a minimum of a month

When beginning a smoothie diet, it requires a lot of time. However, if you remain on it for a month at least, the diet becomes second nature automatically

You want the body to call for further smoothies, like the coffee cup, every day, and even more than once a day.

A month is everything you need to achieve a balanced lifestyle and feel and look so amazing that you would never go without the smoothie for a day.

Agree to a modification

Only when present on the opposite side then you see the elegance of change.

But, when thinking about the nice things on the other end lies of the smoothie plan, be accountable, chat about it, and ask for system help/support.

You ought to be clear regarding the conclusions. Vague consequences prevent you from achieving your objectives.

List them down if you're ill and note that you want to have an improvement in the smoothie plan.

Be reasonable and have an intention behind the desire to adjust.

Get more involved

Sweat it away, in addition to communicating actively about the smoothie plan.

Working out tends you lose calories, and your fitness and appearance are both improved.

You'll maximize weight reduction and health gain outcomes if you visit the gym only 3 days a week.

For a decent sleep at night

During the night, sleeping well leaves you well relaxed and full of energy.

For weight loss, sleep is important also as it keeps you healthy and avoids high cortisol that is responsible for gaining weight.

Consume more water

To speed up your metabolism and keep healthy the cells, you need to remain hydrated.

End up leaving as many of the unhealthy practices as you can

Dream of consuming alcohol or smoking.

Buy a high-velocity blender.

3.3 Smoothie challenge

There are a variety of factors why you may like to participate in a challenge for a smoothie. Know, we are talking of substituting a smoothie for 1 meal a day, most possibly lunch or breakfast. Below are some excellent arguments for taking part in a challenge for smoothies:

Smoothies are an ideal way to introduce to the diet a vast variety of essential nutrients. You will use several different plants in a smoothie, including vegetables, fruit, nuts, seeds, and whole grains. Power from plants.

Smoothies will assist if you have difficulty consuming the required amount of fresh vegetables and fruits in a day.

Smoothies ease healthier eating. There is no cooking involved, only a fast blend, and you've got a complete, healthy, nutritious smoothie.

Smoothies have built-in management of sections. Replacing food with a smoothie will benefit if you have an issue with overeating.

The correct (not the kind filled with sugar) smoothies will combat inflammation and make you feel better.

Smoothie Challenge each smoothie contains:

- Between 350 to 450 calories

- Has 4 + vegetables and fruits servings

- Has no sugar attached

- Is entirely vegan (plant-based)

- Has often more than 10 g of protein

- Just real food ingredients-NO, protein powders

You may expect to consume about 20 types of plant foods in a week only by taking part in the competition. Variety is an essential secret to developing a good immune system and maintaining the body safely. This 31 Days Smoothie Challenge is a perfect starting point to motivate you if you have struggled with getting your healthier eating on line.

Week No. 1

Day No. 1 Banana Peanut Butter Green Smoothie

- Spinach 2 cups

- Banana 1, peeled & frozen

- Natural peanut butter 1 tablespoon

- Vanilla almond milk unsweetened 1 cup

- Cinnamon ¼ to 1/2 teaspoon

- Hulled hemp seeds 3 tablespoons

Instruction

- Place all the ingredients in the blender, mix them until smooth, and then drink

Day   No.   2

Morning glory Smoothie

- Chopped carrots 1 cup

- Apple 1 large, any variety, cored & quartered

- Whole almonds 1/2 ounce (about 1/8 cup)

- Hulled hemp seeds 3 tablespoons

- Pitted dates 2

- Coldwater 1 cup

- Vanilla extract 1/2 tsp

- Cinnamon ¼ to 1/2 tsp

- Ground allspice 1/8 to 1/4 tsp

- Ground cloves 1/8 to 1/4 tsp

Instructions

- Place all the ingredients in the blender, mix them until smooth, and then drink

Day   No.   3

Cucumber melon mint Smoothie

- Spinach 2 cups

- Banana 1, peeled and frozen

- Cubed cantaloupe 1 cup

- Cucumber 1 small, cut in chunks

- Fresh mint leaves 5 to 10

- Coldwater 1/2 cup-1 cup

- Chia   seeds   3   tablespoons

  Instructions

- Place all the ingredients in the blender, mix them until smooth, and then drink

Day   No.   4

Oatmeal Cookie Smoothie

- Rolled oats 1/2 cup

- Raisins 1/4 cup

- Hulled hemp seeds 3 tablespoons

- Vanilla almond milk unsweetened 1 cup

- Vanilla extract 1/2 teaspoon

- Cinnamon ¼ to 1/2 teaspoon

- Ice 1 cup

Instructions

- Place all the ingredients in the blender, mix them until smooth, and then drink

Day   No.   5

Tropical Green smoothie

- Frozen pineapple chunks 1 cup

- Frozen mango chunks 1/2 cup

- Ripe banana 1 (frozen or not)

- Chopped, deveined kale 1 cup

- Hemp seeds 3 tablespoons

- Coldwater 1 cup

Instructions

- Place all the ingredients in the blender, mix them until smooth, and then drink

Day   No.   6

Mango zinger

- Frozen mango chunks 1 cup

- Fresh ginger 1/2 inch, peeled and cut in chunks

- Banana 1, peeled and frozen

- Spinach 2 cups

- Vanilla almond milk unsweetened 1 cup

- Chia seeds 3 tablespoons

- Fresh lime juice 1 tablespoon

Instructions

- Place all the ingredients in the blender, mix them until smooth, and then drink

Day   No.   7

Granny smith and Kale smoothie

- Granny Smith apple 1, cored & quartered

- Chopped kale 1 cup

- Vanilla almond milk unsweetened 1 cup

- Banana 1, peeled and frozen

- Hulled hemp seeds 3 tablespoon

- Ice 1 cup

Instructions

- Place all the ingredients in the blender, mix them until smooth, and then drink

Week No. 2

Day No. 1 Lean Green Machine

- Banana 1, peeled and frozen

- Chopped romaine lettuce 2 cups

- Granny Smith apple 1 large, cored & quartered

- Hemp seeds 3 tablespoons

- Coldwater 1 cup

- Ice

Instructions

- Place all the ingredients in the blender, mix them until smooth, and then drink

Day   No.   2

Blueberry Green Power smoothie

- Frozen blueberries 1 cup

- Chopped parsley 1/2 cup

- Baby spinach 2 cups

- Banana 1, peeled and frozen

- Ground flaxseed 2 tablespoons

- Fresh ginger 1/2 inch, peeled and cut in pieces

- Peanut butter 1-2 tablespoons

- Coldwater 1 cup

Instructions

- Place all the ingredients in the blender, mix them until smooth, and then drink

Day No. 3 Cucumber apple parsley smoothie

- Cucumber 1, cut in chunks

- Apple 1, cored and quartered

- Chopped parsley 1/2 cup

- Pitted dates 2

- 1 lemon juice

- Hulled hemp seeds 3 tablespoons

- Coldwater ½ to 1 cup, to desired consistency

- Ice 1 cup

Instructions

- Place all the ingredients in the blender, mix them until smooth, and then drink

Day No. 4

Avocado-Lada Smoothie

- Frozen pinapple chunks 1 1/2 cups
- Avocado ½
- Baby spinach 2 cups
- Hemp seeds 3 tablespoons
- Coldwater.coconut water 1-1 1/2 cup, to desired consistency

Instructions

- Place all the ingredients in the blender, mix them until smooth, and then drink

Day No. 5

Blueberry Mango Lemonade smoothie

- Frozen blueberries 1/2 cup
- Frozen mango chunks 1/2 cup

- Apple 1 small, cored and quartered

- Chopped romaine lettuce 2 cups

- Chia seeds 3 tablespoons

- 1 lemon juice

- Pitted dates 2

- Vanilla almond milk unsweetened 1 cup

Instructions

- Place all the ingredients in the blender, mix them until smooth, and then drink

Day   No.   6

Chocolate Peanut Butter Smoothie

- Bananas 1 1/2, peeled and frozen

- Unsweetened cocoa powder 3 tablespoons

- Peanut butter 1 tablespoons

- Baby spinach 2 cups

- Ground flaxseed meal 2 tablespoons

- Vanilla almond milk unsweetened 1 cup

- Ice

Instructions

- Place all the ingredients in the blender, mix them until smooth, and then drink

Day   No.   7

Strawberry Beet Dream

- Whole strawberries 1 cup

- Beet 1 small, peeled & diced

- Banana 1, peeled and frozen

- Chia seeds 3 tablespoons

- Dates 2

- Old fashioned oats 1/4 cup

- Coldwater 1 cup

- Ice 1 cup

Instructions

- Place all the ingredients in the blender, mix them until smooth, and then drink

Week No. 3

Day   No.   1

Pumpkin Pie Smoothie

- Pitted dates 3

- Chopped walnuts 1/8 cup

- Rolled oats 1/4 cup

- Pumpkin puree 1 (15 ounces) can

- Pumpkin pie spice 1 tsp

- Vanilla extract 1/2 tsp

- Ground flaxseed meal 1 tablespoon

- Vanilla almond milk unsweetened ½ to 3/4 cup

- Ice 1 cup of

- Stevia (optional)

Instructions

- Place all the ingredients in the blender, mix them until smooth, and then drink

Day   No.   2

Vitamin C power smoothie

- Banana 1/2, frozen

- Orange 1, peel & pith removed & segmented

- Kiwi fruit 1, peeled

- Baby spinach 2 cups

- Lite canned coconut milk 3/4 cup

- Hulled hemp seeds 3 tablespoons

- Ice 1 cup

Instructions

- Place all the ingredients in the blender, mix them until smooth, and then drink

Day   No.   3

Almond Joy Smoothie

- Banana 1/2, frozen

- Whole almonds 1/4 cup

- Pitted dates 2

- Baby spinach 1 cups

- Lite canned coconut milk 3/4 cup

- Unsweetened cocoa powder 2 tablespoons

- Ice 1 cup

- Stevia (optional)

Instructions

- Place all the ingredients in the blender, mix them until smooth, and then drink

Day No. 4 Apple Peanut Butter Green smoothie

- Apple 1 large, cored and quartered

- Banana 1, frozen

- Pitted dates 2

- Swiss chard 1 cup

- Natural peanut butter 1 tablespoon

- Chia seeds 1 tablespoon

- Coldwater 1 cup

- Ice 1 cup

Instructions

- Place all the ingredients in the blender, mix them until smooth, and then drink

Day   No.   5

Next Level Green Smoothie

- Apple 1 large, cored & quartered

- Frozen pineapple 1 cup

- Frozen mango 1/2 cup

- Celery stalk 1, cut in pieces

- Swiss chard 1 cup

- Fresh ginger 1/2 inch, peeled and diced

- Hemp seeds 3 tablespoons

- Coldwater 1 cup

Instructions

- Place all the ingredients in the blender, mix them until smooth, and then drink

Day No. 6 Parsley Spinach Limeade Smoothie

- Baby spinach 1 cup

- Parsley 1/2 cup

- Bananas 1 1/2, frozen

- Whole lime 1, peeled

- Hemp seeds 3 tablespoons

- Small avocado 1/4

- Coldwater 1 cup

- Ice

Instructions

- Place all the ingredients in the blender, mix them until smooth, and then drink

Day   No.   7
Blueberry Chocolate Smoothie

- Frozen blueberries 2 cups

- Pitted dates 2

- Chopped romaine lettuce 2 cups

- Unsweetened cocoa powder 3 tablespoons

- Hemp seeds 3 tablespoons

- Vanilla almond milk unsweetened 1 cup

- Dash cinnamon

Instructions

- Place all the ingredients in the blender, mix them until smooth, and then drink.

Week No. 4

Day No. 1 Minty Watermelon Blueberry Chia

- Watermelon 2 cups

- Frozen blueberries 1 cup

- Large mint leaves 5

- Spinach 2 cups

- Chia seeds 1/4 cup

- 1 cup

Instructions

- Place all the ingredients in the blender, mix them until smooth, and then drink

Day No. 2 Strawberry Banana Oatmeal Smoothie

- Banana 1, peeled and frozen

- Frozen strawberries 1 1/2 cups

- Chopped romaine lettuce 2 cups

- Rolled oats 3/4 cup

- Vanilla almond milk unsweetened 1 cup

- Some ice cubes

Instructions

- Place all the ingredients in the blender, mix them until smooth, and then drink

Day No. 3 Orange Dream Smoothie

- Orange 1 whole, peeled, pith removed, & segmented

- Frozen strawberries 1 cup

- Chopped carrots 1 cup

- Hemp seeds 3 tablespoons

- Walnuts 1/8 cup

- Dash cinnamon

- Coldwater 1/2 cup

- Ice 1 cup

Instructions

- Place all the ingredients in the blender, mix them until smooth, and then drink

Day No. 4 Kiwi Cucumber Smoothie

- Kiwi 2, peeled

- Banana 1, frozen

- Cucumber 1

- Chopped kale 1 cup

- Chia seeds 2 tablespoons

- Ice 1 cup + water, if needed

Instructions

- Place all the ingredients in the blender, mix them until smooth, and then drink

Day No. 5 Spicy Almond ginger smoothie

- Banana 1, frozen

- Fresh ginger 1 inch, peeled and chopped

- Almond butter 2 tablespoons

- Ground flaxseed meal 1/4 cup

- Vanilla almond milk unsweetened 1/2 cup

- Cinnamon 1/4 teaspoon

- (optional) dash cayenne powder

- Ice 1 cup

Instructions

- Place all the ingredients in the blender, mix them until smooth, and then drink

Day No. 6 Orange Chocolate Smoothie

- Whole orange 1, peeled, pith removed, & segmented

- Pitted dates 2

- Unsweetened cocoa powder 3 tablespoons

- Banana 1, frozen

- Hemp seeds 3 tablespoons

- Spinach 2 cups

- Coldwater 1/2 cup to 1 cup

- Ice 1 cup

Instructions

- Place all the ingredients in the blender, mix them until smooth, and then drink

Day No. 7 Va-Va-Vroom energy green smoothie

- Avocado ¼
- Granny smith apple 1, cored and quartered
- Cucumber ½
- Spinach 1 cup
- Chopped romaine 1 cup
- Chopped kale 1 cup
- Banana 1, frozen
- Chia seeds 2 tablespoons
- Coldwater 1 cup
- Ice 1 cup

Instructions

- Place all the ingredients in the blender, mix them until smooth, and then drink

3.4 The Best Smoothie Recipes

1. Apple Coconut Smoothie

- Apple juice 1/4 cup

- Grated coconut 1 pinch or coconut milk 1 tbsp

- Banana 1/2

- Fresh ginger 1/4 teaspoon root peeled

- Ice cubes 2 small

Instructions

- Place all the ingredients in the blender, mix them until smooth, and then drink

2. Apricot Smoothie

- Orange juice 1/4 cup

- Low-fat plain yogurt 1/2 cup

- Peeled, pitted, chopped fresh apricots 1/2 cup

- Honey

Instructions

- Place all the ingredients in a blender. Blend on high speed until smooth

3. Banana Oat Smoothie

- Milk 1 Cup

- Instant Oatmeal 1 Packet, Regular Flavor

- Banana 1 Whole1 Whole, Cut In Chunks

- Orange Juice 1 Cup

Instructions

- Place all the ingredients in the blender, mix them until smooth, and then drink

4.Cantaloupe Berry Smoothie

- Cantaloupe 1/2 – peeled, seeded, cubed

- Plain yogurt 1/2 cup

- Raspberries 1 cup

- White sugar 3 tablespoons

Instructions

- Place all the ingredients in the blender, mix them until smooth, and then drink.

5. Fresh Fruit Smoothie

- Watermelon 1 Cup; Cut Up

- Cantaloupe Or Honeydew 1 Cup

- Pineapple 1 Cup; Cut Up

- Mango 1 Cup; Cut Up

- Strawberries 1 Cup; Halved

- Sugar 1/4 Cup

- Orange Juice 1 Cup
- Crushed Ice

Instruction

- Place all the ingredients in the blender, mix them until smooth, and then drink

6. Healing Smoothie

- Kiwi fruit 1 firm — peeled
- Cantaloupe 1/4 — with skin
- Ripe banana 1

Instructions

- Place all the ingredients in the blender, mix them until smooth, and then drink

7. Kiwi Cooler Smoothie

- Diced fresh kiwi 1 1/2 cups
- Lime sherbet 1 1/2 cups
- Diced ripe banana 1 cup
- Honeydew melon 1 cup

Instructions

- Place all the ingredients in the blender, mix them until smooth, and then drink

8. Lemon Strawberry Yogurt Smoothie

- Nonfat vanilla yogurt 1 cup

- Orange juice 1/2 cup

- Strawberries 1 1/2 cup

- Crushed ice 1/2 cup

- Lemon juice 1 tbsp

- Lemon zest 1/2 tsp

Instructions

- Place all the ingredients in the blender, mix them until smooth, and then drink

9. Mango Tango Smoothie

- Pineapple juice 1 cup

- Orange juice 1 cup

- Frozen banana 1/2 (chunks)

- Pineapple 1 cup sherbet

- Frozen mango 1 1/2 cups sliced

Instructions

* Place all the ingredients in the blender, mix them until smooth, and then drink

10. Melon Madness Smoothie

* Seeded & chopped watermelon 1 1/2 cups
* Seeded & chopped honeydew melon 1 1/2 cups
* 2 limes juice
* Vanilla nonfat yogurt 1 cup
* Ice cubes 1 cup

Instructions

* Place all the ingredients in the blender, mix them until smooth, and then drink

11. Orange Pineapple Coconut Smoothie

* Orange juice 1/4 cup
* Pineapple juice 1/4 cup
* Coconut milk 1 tbsp
* Banana 1/2
* Grated fresh ginger root 1/4 tsp
* Crushed ice 1/2 cup/ice cubes 2 small

Instructions

- Place all the ingredients in the blender, mix them until smooth, and then drink

12. Papaya Raspberry Smoothie

- Frozen banana 1, peeled

- Fresh papaya 1/2

- Raspberries 10-12 (fresh/frozen)

- Water/fruit juice 1/2 cup

Instructions

- Place all the ingredients in the blender, mix them until smooth, and then drink

13. Peach Berry Smoothie

- Nonfat peach yogurt 1 cup

- Peach nectar 3/4 cup

- Raspberries 1/2 cup

- Ripe medium peaches 1 1/2 cup, diced

Instructions

- Place all the ingredients in the blender, mix them until smooth, and then drink

14. Pear Smoothie

- Diced pears 1 1/2 cups

- Peach yogurt 1/2 cup

- Pear nectar 1/2 cup

- Lemon juice 1 tsp.

- Fresh ginger grated 1/4 tsp.

- Ice cubes 3-5

Instructions

- Place all the ingredients in the blender, mix them until smooth, and then drink

15. Quick Morning Smoothie

- Frozen bananas 2

- Sliced frozen peaches 1 cup

- Natural apple juice 1 cup

- Sliced strawberries ½ cup

Instructions

- Place all the ingredients in the blender, mix them until smooth, and then drink

3.5 Reasons why it is much easier to make smoothies than juicing

Blending is good than juicing, especially if you're trying to lose weight

Smoothies can make you fuller for longer, becoming thicker and made of insoluble and soluble fiber.

Here are several explanations below:

Act as food substitutes

A meal is a smoothie of its own, and as a meal substitute, you should drink it. A

meal comprises of macronutrients, as well as vegetables and certain fruit, such as proteins, fats, and carbs.

When they include all these macronutrients and micronutrients, smoothies surely come under the meal parameters.

On the other side, juices are mainly carbohydrates.

Juices do not substitute meals because of the absence of fats and proteins.

Also, the juices are poor in calories.

Anyone who wishes to lose weight must realize that the restriction of calories is counteractive because it slows the metabolism that contributes to weight gain.

Therefore, nuts, coconut milk, Greek yogurt, or nut butter may be applied to smoothies, implying that smoothies are perfect alternatives for meals.

Smoothies will hold you full for longer.

Smoothies include, in addition to the soluble and insoluble fiber, whole food filled with protein.

It takes a long time to digest proteins, so you remain full for a long time, while the fibers slow down the pace at which food flows through your intestine.

Notice that juices are mainly carbohydrates and that they don't have a strong protein content capacity.

As your key protein source, choose flax seeds, peanut butter, Greek yogurt, chia, and hemp seeds.

Smoothies Offer nutrition whole food

For all of the important food classes, a smoothie is a full meal.

Drinking a nutritious smoothie, among other foods, leaves you loaded with fiber, protein, liquids, carbs, fats, minerals, vitamins, and antioxidants.

You will not get entire nutrition consuming juices of insoluble fiber; also, other nutrients extracted from juices.

Sustainable dietary habit are smoothies

While juicing enthusiasts say that drinking fruits and vegetable juices offer relief for the tummy, it doesn't.

A few days' loss of fiber just makes you constipated.

A few days in the juice diet, you often feel tired and lethargic.

Juices often cause long-term metabolic downregulation; on a juice diet, you can quickly add weight.

Even a smoothie cleanse of the short-term improves your metabolism and improves your levels of energy.

This is due to the nutrient abundance of the smoothie.

Drinking two meal substitute smoothies a day, when consumed in the proper manner, helps in weight reduction without hindering the metabolism.

Slower than Juices Smoothies Oxidize

Oxidization is the biggest obstacle to healthy drinks and smoothies.

But smoothies, in comparison to fruits, oxidize at a slower pace.

Studies suggest that, after blending, phytochemicals are higher than after juicing.

This is attributed to the juicing method that makes juices far more susceptible than smoothies to oxidation.

For this, fast-spinning blades are blamed.

Thus, smoothies may be held frozen longer than juices.

Only make sure you keep the smoothie in a tight container, usually a mason jar,

Fiber Slows Absorption of Sugar

Even if you're not obsessed about fruit sugar, you ought to be mindful of the fact that high-sugar vegetables such as carrots and beets are not healthy, concentrated sweeteners.

On the other side, smoothies are abundant with fiber, and they move through the stomach even though strongly loaded with carbohydrates, although the absorption process is slow.

On blood sugar, Blending is easier.

All foods influence blood sugar, but carbohydrates and sugars trigger blood sugar levels to increase, and the effects are not as desirable.

Blood sugar levels are often influenced by proteins and fats but in a positive way.

Studies say that, because of the low glycemic level, proteins and fats minimize blood sugar spikes.

The GI (glycemic index) is the indicator of changes in a healthy person's blood sugar levels after consuming carbohydrate-rich foods.

Carbohydrates are the macronutrients only that induce an acute spike in the blood glucose levels and have a high rating on the GI scale, out of the three major macronutrients, carbohydrates, fats, and proteins.

There is no immediate effect of proteins and fats on blood glucose levels.

Why are we GI cautious?

Well, you find it easier to sustain a healthier weight and even fight diabetes by observing the GI of various foods.

This is helpful because of the need to maintain blood glucose levels down for people who have diabetes.

Sugar increases associated with the urge to sleep after a meal are avoided with the inclusion of fats and proteins to smoothies.

Smoothies Minimize waste from food

That there is minimum waste is one of the reasons why We promote blending.

Juicing leaves nearly half pulp in the trash.

It just makes sense to use food storage strategies that eliminate as much waste as possible in a country where the majority of people reside in poverty.

So, juices are unhealthy?

Despite the reasoning for blending above, juices are not harmful.

You should also mix all smoothies & juices with the correct ingredients to boost your overall wellbeing.

While juicing isn't a big part of your lifestyle, just change it up and drink juices once in a while.

Why?

- Juices and Smoothies increase fruit and vegetable intake.

- They are also liquids as well, and you can quickly assimilate them.

- Even in the smoothie, you need a healthier substitute to the chunky bits, and that's where the juices come in. Keep juicing to a minimum to find a compromise and to remain safe and genuinely consider this an occasional nutritious treat.

As discussed above, juicing affects metabolism by making you starve, particularly as cleanses.

You can lose weight on a 4 out of 5-day juice cleanse, but you're going to starve eventually.

Therefore, long-term weight reduction reliance on juicing would not perform very well.

Juicing's other adverse effects include:

- Deprivation of healthy food fibers

- Juices boost the risk of type II diabetes by supplying a large dose of the readily ingested carbohydrates into the bloodstream.

Conclusion

Smoothies offer a convenient way to consume less and with vital foods to nourish the body. The ideal benefits would result in smart choices of fresh vegetables and fruits and producing your smoothie. All you need is this guide and a blender. As a food substitute or a food supplement, smoothies can drink. Smoothies can be tasty and perfect for both adults and children. Most varieties of vegetables and fruits are simpler to eat in blended form than when prepared. It is simple and fast to make smoothies. The majority of smoothies are available in around 10 mins. It is possible to consume smoothies on the go. They can be made anywhere and anywhere with handheld blenders.- Smoothies are readily digested, which can help alleviate the severity of food cravings.

CPSIA information can be obtained
at www.ICGtesting.com
Printed in the USA
LVHW051814200121
677011LV00028B/950